USMLE STEP 2 CK Infectious Diseases In Your Pocket

✓ Study guide for the USMLE STEP 2 CK exam.
✓ Prepare for your shelf examination.
✓ Be ready for your inpatient rotation.

Gregory J. Fernandez M.D.

First Edition, 2016
Author & Editor: Gregory J. Fernandez, M.D.
Publisher: M.D. Educational Services
Peer Reviewer: Tahira N. Sánchez Muñoz, MD
Book Design: Marie Meyer
Copyediting: Editage Cactus Communications

DISCLAIMER: The author, editor, publisher, and staff members have taken care to confirm the accuracy of the information present in this publication. The context of the books entirety, is believed to be reliable in accordance with the standards accepted at the time of publication. However, readers are encouraged to confirm the information and conduct their own research for clarification of all the information present within this book. No one involved in creating this book is responsible for errors or omissions or for any consequences from application of the information in this book. There is no warranty, expressed or implied, with respect to the completeness or accuracy of the contents of this publication. Neither the editor, nor the author assumes any liability for any injury and/or damage to persons or property arising from the content of this publication. Application of this information in a particular situation remains the professional responsibility of the practitioner; the clinical treatments or information described and recommended may not be considered absolute and universal recommendations. It is the responsibility of the health care provider to ascertain the FDA status of each drug used or device planned for use in their clinical practice. The purpose of this books, is to be used as a study guide for medical examinations. Please consult with attending physicians for any medical decisions.

Copyright © 2016 by Gregory J. Fernandez M.D. All rights reserved. This book or any portion thereof may not be reproduced or used in any manner whatsoever without the express written permission of the publisher except for the use of brief quotations in a book review. Printed in the United States of America, 2016, M.D. Educational Services, Santa Fe, New Mexico. Contact us at md.educational.services@hotmail.com.

ISBN-13: 978-1532855153
ISBN-10: 153285515X

> *This book is gratefully dedicated to my wife. Thank you for your support and always being there for me. Thank you for your kindness, your devotion, and your endless selflessness support. I love you... Thank you mother, father, step-mother, brothers, friends, and family for all your encouragement and endless love. Best of luck to all the medical dreamers, the road is long and I hope my book helps you through this journey. All the best...*

How to Use
"Infectious Diseases In Your Pocket"

Infectious Diseases In Your Pocket is a study guide for the USMLE STEP 2 CK exam that you can also use to prepare for your shelf examination and to get ready for your inpatient rotation. It is part of a series, each dealing with a different subject or sub-specialty, focusing on vital clinical knowledge.

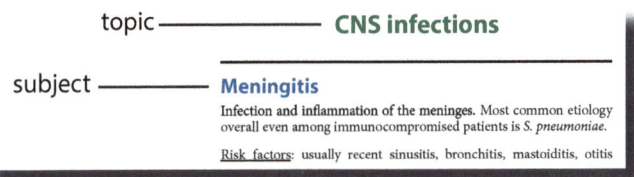

The subjects and topics within infectious diseases are called out in large, colored type. These items are also included in the Table of Contents for ease of access.

Many subjects also contain sub-subjects that are also called out in bold, blue type either as bulleted items or in-line with the text, as appropriate. They are all referenced in the index.

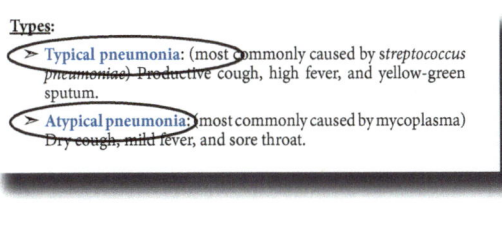

Presentation of clinical history and physical exam (Hx/PE), step-by-step diagnosis, and treatment plan are indicated by bold red headings.

> **Hx/PE**: Rash begins on face and neck and spreads downward (sparing palms and soles). Might present with "strawberry tongue" and high fevers.
>
> **Diagnosis**: CBC (lymphocytosis), ESR (elevated), CRP (elevated), throat culture (positive), and elevated antistreptolysin O titer (ASO titer).
>
> **Treatment**: Amoxicillin or macrolides (azithromycin) as alternative (if allergic).

Procedures, triads, pathology, medications, antibodies and findings are called out in bold text. These items are also included in the index.

> - **ELISA test** (high sensitivity) followed by **Western blot** (high specificity) for confirmation in adults or children >18 months old. Western blot has a higher false positive if <18 months of age.

Reflexes, signs and maneuvers are shown in purple text.

> ✓ If patient is allergic to penicillin and <u>not</u> pregnant, can use doxycycline or tetracycline for 14 days
>
> ✓ Treatment of syphilis can cause **Jarisch-Herxheimer reaction** (flu-like symptoms). If develops, usually self-limiting but can use aspirin.

Mnemonics and key words are shown in orange text.

> endocarditis.
>
> **Hx/PE**: Rash begins on face and neck and spreads downward (sparing palms and soles). Might present with "strawberry tongue" and high fevers.
>
> **Diagnosis**: CBC (lymphocytosis), ESR (elevated), CRP (elevated),

And, finally, for the avoidance of doubt, circumstances that amount to a medical emergency are flagged with a warning.

> *Neisseria gonorrhoeae* **conjunctivitis**
>
> **Medical emergency** that can lead to blindness. Usually presents around day 3 post-partum.
>
> **Diagnosis**: Gram stain (diplococcal) or PCR.

Infectious Diseases In Your Pocket

Infectious Diseases
Table of Contents

Pneumonias 3
   Pneumonia Overview 3

Upper respiratory infections 6
   Sinusitis 6
   Acute otitis media (AOM) 7
   Otitis externa (swimmer's ear) 8
   Acute pharyngitis 9
   Peritonsillar abscess 10
   Retropharyngeal abscess 11
   Influenza A, B, and C 11
   Infectious mononucleosis 12
   Scarlet fever 14

CNS infections 14
   Meningitis 14
   Citrobacter koseri 17
   Encephalitis 18
   Brain abscess 19
   Cavernous sinus thrombosis 20

**Human immuno-
deficiency virus** 21
   Human immunodeficiency virus
   (HIV) 21

HIV-related infections 24
   Pneumocystis jiroveci pneumonia
   (PJP) 24
   Toxoplasmosis 24
   Mycobacterium avium complex
   (MAC) 25
   Cytomegalovirus (CMV) 26
   Progressive multifocal leukoen-
   cephalopathy (PML) 27
   Tuberculosis (TB) 27
   Cryptococcal meningitis 30
   Oropharyngeal candidiasis 30
   Coccidioidomycosis 31
   Blastomycosis 32
   Histoplasmosis 32
   Aspergillus 33

Tick bites 34
   Lyme disease 34
   Rocky Mountain spotted fever
   (*Rickettsia rickettsii*) 35

Sexually transmitted diseases ... 36
   Chlamydia 36
   Gonorrhea 37
   Syphilis (*Treponema pallidum*) ... 37
   Haemophilus ducreyi 39
   Human papillomavirus (condylo-
   mata acuminate) 39
   Pelvic inflammatory disease 40

Genitourinary infections 41
   Urinary tract infections 41
   Pyelonephritis 43
   Group A hemolytic streptococcus
   (GAS) 44
   Group B hemolytic streptococcus
   (GBS) 44
   Nocardia asteroides 44
   Actinomyces israelii 45

Sepsis 45
   Sepsis 45

Protozoan 46
   Malaria 46

Animal bites 47
   Rabies 47

Ocular infections 48
   Bacterial conjunctivitis 48
   Viral conjunctivitis 49
   Neisseria gonorrhoeae
   conjunctivitis 49
   Chlamydia trachomatis
   conjunctivitis 50
   Orbital cellulitis 50
   Corneal abrasion 50

Infectious Diseases
Table of Contents, cont'd

Chalazion 51
Hordeolum (stye) 51

Endocarditis 52
Infective endocarditis (IE) 52

Osteomyelitis 53
Osteomyelitis 53
Anthrax 55
Botulinum toxin 56
Index, cont'd. 58

Pneumonias

Pneumonia Overview

"Pneumonia" is a broad term referring to inflammation of the lungs which may be caused by many factors. It frequently starts as an upper respiratory tract infection that develops into a lower respiratory tract infection.

Types:

- Typical pneumonia: (most commonly caused by *streptococcus pneumoniae*) Productive cough, high fever, and yellow-green sputum.
- Atypical pneumonia: (most commonly caused by mycoplasma) Dry cough, mild fever, and sore throat.

Common etiology by age:

- 0–6 weeks (Group B streptococcus [GBS]).
- 6 weeks–18 years (RSV).
- 18 years–40 years (mycoplasma).
- >40 years (*S. pneumoniae*).

Note:

- ✓ *S. pneumoniae* is the most common overall cause of typical pneumonia.
- ✓ Mycoplasma pneumonia is the most common overall cause of atypical pneumonia (in healthy patients).

Hx/PE:

- Typical pneumonia: physical exam includes localized dullness to percussion, localized tactile fremitus, fever, chills, cough, night sweats, chest pain, and difficulty breathing.
- Atypical pneumonia: physical exam can be similar but without localized findings; usually physical findings are bilateral or can be unilateral.

Diagnosis:

- Best initial diagnostic test is a chest x-ray.

- **Typical bacteria** (lobular consolidation).
- **Atypical bacteria** or fungus infection (diffused bilateral interstitial infiltrates).
- <u>Community-acquired pneumonia</u> (bacterial) classically shows lobular consolidation of one segmental lobe.
- CBC (leukocytosis), electrolytes, ABG (hypoxia), NP swab, sputum culture (most accurate test), blood culture (if evidence of sepsis), and chest radiography (is diagnostic).
- Mycoplasma pneumonia: can use cold agglutinins (low specificity and sensitivity), which can be helpful in confirming diagnosis.

Note: first round of orders for pneumonia are oxygen, oximeter, ABG, and chest radiography.

Treatment:

- Outpatient: oral antibiotics (if uncomplicated), most commonly azithromycin (Z-pack), clarithromycin, or doxycycline.
- Inpatient: always use IV antibiotics. Common first choice is IV macrolides with IV 2nd or 3rd generation cephalosporins.
- Toddlers with community acquired pneumonia: outpatient amoxicillin.
- Influenza A or B: use oseltamivir, zanamivir, or peramivir (best if given within 48 hours of onset).
- Recurrent bacterial infections: consider quantitative measurement of serum immunoglobulin levels.

Note: inpatient treatment required if, multiple risk factors, >65 years of age, chronic obstructive pulmonary disease, heart disease, diabetes, immunosuppression, alcoholism, or respiratory failure.

Treatment types:

Aspiration pneumonia (anaerobes)

Treatment:

- Clindamycin (if uncomplicated).
- If hospitalized and/or elderly patient, use clindamycin plus levofloxacin.

Neonate PNA (GBS)
Treatment: Amoxicillin (best choice).

Cystic fibrosis (cover *Pseudomonas*).
Treatment: Ciprofloxacin or cefepime

Post-viral (*Staphylococcus aureus*).
Treatment: Oxacillin.

Atypical: Mycoplasma (bilateral findings).
Treatment: Azithromycin or fluoroquinolones.

Community-acquired (*S. pneumoniae*)
Treatment: Azithromycin or doxycycline (if resistant). Can also use fluoroquinolones.

Critically ill or no improvement after 48 hours.
Treatment: Vancomycin or linezolid.

Hospital-acquired (cover *S. pseudomonas*).
Treatment: Cefepime, ceftazidime, tobramycin, piperacillin, and vancomycin or linezolid. Can add fluoroquinolones.

Alcoholics (*S. pneumoniae*, followed by *Klebsiella* "currant jelly sputum").
Treatment: Ceftriaxone.

Legionellosis (air conditioning).
Treatment: Azithromycin or doxycycline.

Fun facts:

- Do not give doxycycline for children younger than 8 years of age.
- If older teen and bilateral findings give azithromycin (most common bacteria will be mycoplasma pneumoniae).
- If obstructive disease (cystic fibrosis or bronchiectasis), <u>add</u> pseudomonal, staphylococcal, and anaerobic coverage.
- Hospital-acquired methicillin-resistant *S. aureus* (MRSA) should always be treated with IV vancomycin.
- Patients with aspiration risks (stroke patients, amyotrophic lateral sclerosis [ALS], Alzheimer's disease, dementia, and sedation) will need a **speech and swallow study** and be placed on aspiration precautions.
- Aspiration pneumonia is different from **aspiration pneumonitis**. Aspiration pneumonia requires antibiotics, and aspiration pneumonitis does not.

Upper respiratory infections

Sinusitis

Most commonly caused by viral infections and typically affect the maxillary sinuses. If bacterial etiology, S. pneumoniae is the most common.

➤ Acute sinusitis: <1 month.
  Most common cause of <u>acute</u> sinusitis is an upper respiratory infection.
➤ Chronic sinusitis: >3 months.
  Most common cause of <u>chronic</u> sinus infections is a septal deformity.

Diagnosis:
- Clinical diagnosis:
  - Bacterial infection: physical exam findings --> positive transillumination, tooth pain, sinus pain, fever, and rhinorrhea.

- Viral infections are usually mild and last only about a week.
- Consider bacterial infection when high fever, unilateral congestion, or last longer than the usual course of a viral infection of 10 days.

If symptoms continue after treatment or ≥ 3 months consider sinus radiography, followed by sinus culture (most accurate), and maxillary CT scan.

Treatment:
- Viral sinusitis: self-limiting and treat symptoms with nasal decongestants (Afrin), systemic anti-histamines, and NSAIDs are helpful.
  - If not resolved within 10 days need to consider bacterial sinusitis.
- Acute bacterial sinusitis: start with amoxicillin alone (3-7 days). If not better after 7 days consider amoxicillin/clavulanate. Alternative medications are azithromycin or 2nd generation cephalosporins.
  - Studies still support 10-day treatment for children.
- Chronic bacterial sinusitis: amoxicillin/clavulanate for 21 days plus administer intranasal corticosteroids, nasal decongestants, and oral anti-histamines.
- Severe, recurrent, or chronic: consider surgical intervention. Referral to an otolaryngologist may be indicated.

Note: if recurrent bacterial sinusitis infections, rule out septal deformity and immunodeficiency's (order serum immunoglobulin levels).

Acute otitis media (AOM)

An inflammatory disease of the middle ear that is usually precipitated by an upper respiratory tract infection. Most common agents are S. pneumoniae, nontypeable haemophilus influenzae, moraxella catarrhalis, RSV, and parainfluenza. An important risk factor is exposure to second hand cigarette smoke in children.

Hx/PE: Erythema of tympanic membrane, immobility of the tympanic membrane (most sensitive), retraction, bulging, and secretions.

Diagnosis: Clinical diagnosis (otoscopic examination or pneumatic otoscope). Most accurate test is **tympanocentesis**.

Treatment:

- Acute in children: amoxicillin 80–90 mg/kg/10 days. Usually see results in 3 days; if no results, switch antibiotics.
- Resistant/recurrent: combination of amoxicillin with clavulanic acid.
- Chronic: consider tympanic tubes (order hearing test).
    - Consider tympanic tubes in individuals who have 3 or more episodes of acute otitis media in 6 months or 4 or more in a year.
    - If evidence of hearing loss on audiometry, conduct **myringotomy** (incision of tympanic membrane to release fluid) and insert tympanostomy tubes.
- Fluid may persist in middle ear for up to 3 months after treatment, which requires watchful waiting. If last longer than 3 months then consider further therapy.

Symptomatic relief: decongestants or intranasal steroids can be helpful.

Note:

✓ Patients have increased risk of recurrent AOM even after treatment.

✓ Remember that patients might have persistent fluid in lungs for 3 months after treatment, but this does not mean they need further work-up or treatment.

Otitis externa (swimmer's ear)

Infection of external auditory canal most common secondary to infections caused by pseudomonas, which loves water.

Hx/PE: Erythema and drainage of external ear with pain on moving or pulling on tragus/pinna.

Diagnosis:

- Clinical diagnosis or swab culture (if suspicion of etiology other than pseudomonas).

- If appears toxic, perform head CT scan to rule out osteomyelitis (**malignant otitis externa**).
- If bone involvement, bone biopsy is the most accurate diagnostic tool; however, best initial test is MRI of the head.

Treatment:
- Cleaning and debridement.
- Topical fluoroquinolone and steroid eardrops (helps with itching and inflammation).
- Acetic acid and drying agents can help eliminate infection.
- If severe or not cured topically, will need IV antibiotics.

Note: After a few days of treatment, patient can return to daily activities including swimming.

Acute pharyngitis

Most commonly caused by viral infections (40-80%), with adenovirus being the most common. However, the most common bacterial agent is Group A streptococcus.(GAS) Risk of developing rheumatic fever, post-streptococcal glomerulonephritis, sinusitis, otitis media, mastoiditis, and peritonsillar abscess.

➢ **Viral pharyngitis**: pharyngeal erythema, no exudate, hoarseness, dry cough, rhinorrhea, and mild fever.
➢ **Bacterial pharyngitis**: pharyngeal erythema, "**tonsillar exudate**," cervical lymphadenopathy, high fever, and sore throat.

Diagnosis:
- Most often a clinical diagnosis.
- Best initial test is rapid streptococcal test (if rapid strep test is positive, no need to obtain throat culture).
  - If positive rapid streptococcal test, prescribe antibiotics.
  - If rapid streptococcal test is negative and continued high suspicion because of positive physical exam, start treatment with antibiotics. Obtain a throat culture; if culture returns negative, stop antibiotics, and if culture returns positive, continue antibiotics.

Infectious Diseases In Your Pocket

- Confirmatory tests: rapid streptococcal test, NP swab, and possible throat culture (if no improvement with standard treatment or perform after a negative rapid strep test, to confirm presents of infection).

Note:
- ✓ Basically, a rapid strep test is performed first, followed by a throat culture, if needed.
- ✓ If clinical diagnosis of bacterial infection even after negative rapid strep, start antibiotics, but confirm with throat culture (specific).

Treatment:
- Viral pharyngitis: fluids, rest, salt-water gargles, tea, vitamin C, Echinacea lozenges, NSAIDs, and antitussives.
- Bacterial pharyngitis: if GAS, oral penicillin V for 10 days or 1 dose of penicillin G intramuscularly. GAS is treated to avoid acute rheumatic fever (can lead to endocarditis).
- Azithromycin is the alternative if allergic if the patient is allergic to penicillin.

Peritonsillar abscess

Considered to be an abscess of the tonsils, which is a collection of pus posterior to the tonsil. Suspected post-pharyngitis with persistent fever and worsening sore throat despite treatment.

Hx/PE: Dysphagia, fever, and uvula deviates to unaffected side.

Diagnosis: CBC, electrolytes, ESR, rapid streptococcal test, NP swab, sputum culture, and intra-oral ultrasound. If surgical drainage is performed, obtain a culture of the flue.

Treatment:
- Oral or IV antibiotics (clindamycin) in combination with penicillin G and surgical drainage (often needed).
- Be aware of the need to secure the airway if obstruction is suspected.
- If severe obstruction or dysphagia, the patient might require surgical removal of tonsils (**tonsillectomy**).

Note: surgical drainage and antibiotics should be used for almost all abscesses, but is not always required in the case of hepatic abscess.

Retropharyngeal abscess

An abscess located in the posterior pharyngeal wall. Suspect this in cases where the patient has with history of recent pharyngitis and extended course of infection despite conservative treatment.

Hx/PE: Stiff neck, dysphagia, and pain on palpation of neck area.

Diagnosis:
- CBC, ESR, rapid streptococcal test, sputum culture, and lateral films confirm diagnosis.
- Neck CT is the definitive diagnostic test.

Treatment:
- IV antibiotics (clindamycin) and surgical drainage.
- Consider tonsillectomy.
- If airway obstruction, secure airway or perform intubation (rarely needed).

Influenza A, B, and C

Orthomyxovirus (RNA virus). Classified based on glycoproteins (hemagglutinin and neuraminidase).

➤ **Genetic drift**: small gradual mutations caused mainly by point mutations.

➤ **Genetic shift**: major changes caused mainly by frame shifts and genetic re-assortment.

Hx/PE: Common during change of seasons with cough, chills, mild fevers, fatigue, and myalgia.

Diagnosis:
- **Rapid influenza diagnostic test** (RIDT) or NP swab (can detect both viruses and bacteria).

- Definitive diagnosis is by throat culture.
- Leukopenia and low platelets are common findings with viral infections.

Note: With NP swab, ask patient to first cough; then place head back to insert cotton swab into nose.

Treatment:

- Treat symptoms: rest, fluids, vitamin C, echinacea lozenges, NSAIDs, and antitussives.
- Oseltamivir or zanamivir (most effective if administered within 2 days and can shorten course by 1–2 days). Required if patient is hospitalized, high-risk patients, or lower respiratory symptoms.
- Amantadine is <u>only</u> effective against influenza A.
- If 48 hours have passed or illness is mild, or mild illness, provide supportive therapy.

Vaccinations:

➤ <u>Intramuscular (IM) influenza vaccination</u> (killed vaccination): the CDC recommends that everyone 6 months and older should get a yearly influenza vaccination.

- High risk patients are patients <18 years of age, >50 years of age, diabetes, heart disease, COPD, comorbidities, asthma, immunosuppressed, health care workers, or pregnancy. Can be administered as early as 6 months of age.

➤ **Intranasal influenza vaccination** (live vaccination): can be administered to healthy individuals aged 2–49 years. Do **not** administer if immunosuppressed, pregnant, or younger than 2 years of age.

Infectious mononucleosis "kissing disease"

Acute EBV infection typically presents in young adults from exchange of saliva or body fluids. Commonly misdiagnosed because of presentation with pharyngitis and tonsillar exudate that resembles bacterial pharyngitis.

Complications:
- CNS infections (encephalitis).
- Patients with splenic rupture (<0.5%) cannot participate in competitive sports until negative radiological studies or negative physical exam.
- Lymphadenopathy should regress in about 2-4 weeks; if persistent consider biopsy.
- Can develop secondary streptococcal pharyngitis.
- Fulminant hepatic necrosis.
- Autoimmune hemolytic anemia (Coombs +).
- Oral squamous cell cancer.
- Pericarditis.
- Pneumonia.

Hx/PE: Fever, fatigue, pharyngitis, lymphadenopathy, tonsillar exudates, and splenomegaly.

Diagnosis:
- CBC (thrombopenia with lymphocytosis).
- Test of choice is **monospot test** (screens for **heterophile antibody**), which can be negative in the first few weeks.
- Most sensitive and specific diagnostic study is IgM **EBV antibody to viral capsid antigen**.
- Can consider abdominal ultrasound (controversial) to observe splenomegaly.

Note: If patient also presents with rash and diarrhea, human immunodeficiency virus (HIV) needs to be ruled out. HIV infection and mononucleosis have similar symptoms. Also consider the possibility of lymphomas (neck lymphadenopathy).

Treatment:
- Supportive care (self-limited) such as fluids, rest, and NSAIDs.
- Some studies suggest valacyclovir used for EBV can decrease severity.
- Consider IV steroids if closing airway (rare).

Preventions:

- If needed, treat underlying bacterial pharyngitis, pericarditis, pneumonia, and anemia.
- Most fatal complication is splenic rupture (avoid contact sports).

Note: if misdiagnosed and treated with ampicillin for streptococcal pharyngitis, will cause maculopapular rash (secondary to circulating immune complexes). In this case, discontinue antibiotics.

Scarlet fever

An infectious disease that can lead to glomerulonephritis and endocarditis.

Hx/PE: Rash begins on face and neck and spreads downward (sparing palms and soles). Might present with "strawberry tongue" and high fevers.

Diagnosis: CBC (lymphocytosis), ESR (elevated), CRP (elevated), throat culture (positive), and elevated antistreptolysin O titer (ASO titer).

Treatment: Amoxicillin or macrolides (azithromycin) as alternative (if allergic).

Vaccination: no vaccines are currently available against *S. pyogenes* infection.

CNS infections

Meningitis

Infection and inflammation of the meninges. Most common etiology overall even among immunocompromised patients is *S. pneumoniae*.

Risk factors: usually recent sinusitis, bronchitis, mastoiditis, otitis media, or pneumonia infections. CNS surgery (*S. aureus*) vs. CNS shunts (epididymitis).

Etiology by age group: "rule of 6s."

➢ 0–6 months: GBS.

➢ 6 months–6 years: *S. pneumoniae* (gram-positive diplococci).

➢ 6 years–60 years: *N. meningitidis* (gram-negative diplococci).

➢ >60 years: *S. pneumoniae*.

Note: GBS is otherwise known as *S. agalactiae* (gram-positive cocci in pairs and chains).

Hx/PE: Headache, fever, neck stiffness, photophobia, petechial rash (common in N*eisseria meningitidis*), seizures, altered mental status, nausea, and vomiting. Infection secondary to *S. pneumoniae* does not present with petechial rash. Can present with positive **Brudzinski's sign** and **Kernig's sign**.

Diagnosis:

- Physical exam and CBC (leukocytosis), ESR (elevated), and CRP (elevated).
- Bacterial meningitis: treatment should not be delayed, lumbar puncture should be attempted first.
  - However, if papilledema, neurofocal findings, seizures, immunocompromised state, stroke, or altered mental status, perform head CT scan first. If CT scan is normal, perform a lumbar puncture.
- Perform a lumbar puncture to confirm diagnosis and start treatment immediately.
  - Order CSF sample (most specific test): glucose, gram stain, cell count, proteins, RBCs, WBCs, and open pressure.
- Blood culture (rule out sepsis).
- **Fever of unknown origin** is most commonly caused by infection.

Extended diagnosis:

➢ Bacterial meningitis: CSF with neutrophil-predominant pleocytosis.

➢ Viral meningitis: CSF with lymphocyte-predominant pleocytosis.

➢ CSF differentials:

- Bacterial: increased PNM, increased proteins, increased open pressure, and decreased glucose.
- Viral: increased lymphocytes, normal glucose, increased proteins, and increased open pressure.
- Fungal: increased lymphocytes, mild decrease in glucose, increased proteins, and increased open pressure.
- Atypical bacterial: increased lymphocytes, mild decrease in glucose, increased proteins, and increased open pressure.
- Subarachnoid hemorrhage: increased RBCs.
- Herpes encephalitis: increased RBCs.
- Multiple sclerosis: increased IgG (oligoclonal bands).
- Guillain-Barre: increased proteins.
- Pseudotumor: increased open pressure.
- * No elevation in proteins in CSF almost excludes meningitis.

Treatment:
- Bacterial meningitis: requires immediate IV antibiotics. Antibiotics can be administered up to 2 hours before lumbar puncture. However, if stable best to get LP first (if no contraindications).
- Dexamethasone (decreases mortality) can be started before or during the first dose of antibiotics.
- Dexamethasone is not helpful for *N. meningitidis*.
- If caused by *N. meningitidis*, isolate patient; restraints may be necessary if they if resist treatment.
- Viral meningitis: supportive care (fluids and analgesics). Usually self-limiting.
- Syphilis meningitis: IV penicillin for 14 days. Desensitization if allergic to penicillin.
- Lyme meningitis: IV ceftriaxone.
- Cryptococcal meningitis: IV amphotericin B.
- Rocky Mountain spotted fever: IV doxycycline.
- Adult TB meningitis: standard medications for 9 months instead of 6 months, plus ADD dexamethasone.
- Neonate TB meningitis: treat for 12 months.

Common meningitis treatments based on age:
- <1 month: amoxicillin plus cefotaxime or gentamicin.
- >1 month to adulthood: IV ceftriaxone plus vancomycin.
- >50 years: IV ceftriaxone plus vancomycin and ampicillin or gentamicin.

Fun Facts:
- Close contact is defined as direct contact with oral secretions, such as an intimate partner, people who share cups or utensils, or a health care provider who intubated the patient.
  - If patient is diagnosed with meningococcal meningitis, administer prophylaxis to close contacts with rifampin (4 doses orally) or IM ceftriaxone (preferred if the exposed person is pregnant). Also need to place patient in respiratory isolation.
- Rifampin: only prophylaxis for *N. meningitides* and *Haemophilus influenzae* type b; not *S. pneumoniae*.
- Ampicillin is added for patients <1 month or >50 years of age to cover for listeria. Often, a Gram stain fails to show the organism.
- Side effects of gentamycin: "NOT": nephrotoxic, ototoxic, and teratogenic.
  - Patient receiving gentamycin need to have a hearing test, urine hCG, and BUN/Cr ratio measured before and after treatment. Measure trough during treatment.
- Vancomycin and levofloxacin need to be renally dosed.
- Headaches are a side effect of lumbar punctures, and patient should lie down to decrease symptoms.
- If resistant to vancomycin, use linezolid, which can cause thrombocytopenia.

Citrobacter koseri

Can cause bacterial meningitis in neonates, which often presents as a brain abscess.

Diagnosis: Head CT scan or MRI.

Treatment:
- 3rd generation cephalosporins and aminoglycosides for 4 weeks.
- Abscess will frequently need drainage.

Encephalitis

Encephalitis is inflammation of the brain tissue. Most commonly caused by HSV, enterovirus, arbovirus, and cytomegalovirus (CMV). More common in AIDs patients, children, and elderly populations.

Hx/PE: Fever, headache, nausea, vomiting, *altered mental status, seizure, focal neurological deficits, and "accentuated DTRs." Focal finding is more specific here, compared with meningitis.

Diagnosis:
- First, head CT scan before lumbar puncture, because the patient will usually have altered mental status. Do not perform a lumbar puncture before head CT scan, if altered mental status, focal findings, papillary edema, or seizures.
- Brain MRI offers more resolution for soft tissue inflammation than head CT scan.
- Lumbar puncture (CSF analysis):
  - HSV: often increased RBCs.
  - Fungal or amebic: low glucose, high proteins, increased pressure, and increased WBCs.
  - Tuberculosis: special test is culture for acid fast.
  - Cryptococcus: special test is India ink or cryptococcal antigen.
  - Trypanosomes: special test is PCR or Giemsa stain.
  - HSV, CMV, EBV, and varicella-zoster virus: special test is PCR.
- Brain biopsy is <u>not</u> needed here.

Note: if negative India ink stain, which might only be diagnostic up to 75% of the time, and high suspicion of cryptococcal meningitis, order a cryptococcal antigen from CSF (more specific).

Treatment:
- HSV encephalitis: start empirical treatment with IV acyclovir; do not delay for diagnostic studies if clinically suspected. If resistant to acyclovir, use foscarnet.
- CMV encephalitis: ganciclovir.
- Rocky Mountain fever encephalitis: doxycycline.
- Lyme disease encephalitis: doxycycline or 3rd generation cephalosporins.

Note: can use steroids (decrease brain swelling) and seizure prophylaxis (phenytoin).

Brain abscess

Most common pathology causing brain abscesses are streptococcal, staphylococcal, polymicrobial, and anaerobe infections.

➢ Direct spread: secondary to sinusitis, otitis media, mastoiditis, or URI.
➢ Direct inoculation: trauma or neurosurgery.
➢ Hematogenous spread: blood.

Hx/PE: Dull and constant headache (most common), focal neurologic deficit, seizures, and altered mental status. Look out for focal findings and papillary edema.

Diagnosis:
- CBC, electrolytes, blood culture, ESR, and CRP.
- First test: head CT scan with contrast ("ring-enhancing lesion") and MRI (higher sensitivity for early abscesses and abscesses in posterior fossa).
  - Ring enhancing lesion secondary to fibrous capsule.
  - Focal infection of brain parenchyma.
  - Rule out brain tumor (similar presentation).
  - Can look similar to toxoplasmosis.
- Most accurate test is aspiration biopsy.

Note: <u>no</u> lumbar puncture for brain abscess because might cause **brain herniation**.

Treatment:

- IV antibiotics: ceftriaxone + metronidazole or clindamycin and +/- vancomycin.
- Surgical drainage: if >2 cm and/or need culture.
- Dexamethasone or IV mannitol, if increased intracranial pressure.

Note: viral infections are never encountered in brain abscess.

Clindamycin:

- Commonly used for aspiration pneumonia, lung abscess, brain abscess, necrotizing fasciitis, oral infections, and neck infections.
- <u>Side effects</u>: can cause growth of *Clostridium difficile* in GI tract, usually takes a couple weeks to develop.

Cavernous sinus thrombosis (CST)

A blood clot within the cavernous sinus. Most commonly secondary to bacterial thrombosis (Staphylococcus aureus and Streptococcus). The cause is usually from a spreading infection from the nose, sinuses, ears, or teeth.

Hx/PE: Headache, fever, altered mental status, eye swelling, proptosis, papilledema, ptosis, mydriasis, and blurry vision.

Diagnosis:

- CBC, ESR, blood culture (if septic), and LP (is necessary to rule out meningitis).
- Head CT scan or MRI with pituitary protocol.

Treatment:

- IV antibiotics, high dose corticosteroids (controversial), and thrombolytics (controversial).
    - <u>MSSA</u>: use nafcillin or oxacillin <u>plus</u> third-/fourth-generation cephalosporin.

- MRSA: use vancomycin plus third-/fourth-generation cephalosporin.

Human immunodeficiency virus

Human immunodeficiency virus (HIV)

A retrovirus that destroys CD+4 and T-lymphocytes. Can present with an increase in viral load and decrease in CD4+ count; which means worse prognosis.

- CD4+ count: indicates degree of immunosuppression and guides prophylaxis and therapy.
- Viral load: rate of disease and response to anti-retroviral therapy.

HIV in children:

- Can present with failure to thrive, developmental delay, fever, oral thrush, lymphadenopathy, and recurrent infections.
- Risk of HIV transmission from mother to newborn:
    - 25% risk if no anti-retroviral therapy or cesarean delivery given.
    - 8.0% risk if given anti-retroviral therapy alone.
    - 2.0% risk if both antiretroviral therapy and scheduled cesarean delivery (always encourage cesarean unless viral load <1,000).

Hx/PE: First presents with thrombocytopenia and flu-like or mononucleosis-like symptoms. If have flu-like symptoms with rash and diarrhea, consider HIV.

Diagnosis:

- **ELISA test** (high sensitivity) followed by **Western blot** (high specificity) for confirmation in adults or children >18 months old. Western blot has a higher false positive if <18 months of age.
- Rapid HIV tests now available.

- HIV RNA PCR assay provides <u>definitive</u> diagnosis.
- Order HIV genotype (can help determine treatment).

<u>Screening</u>: can consider screening in any individual despite risk factors. However, highly consider screening if history of tuberculosis, syphilis, male homosexual contact, IV drug use, viral hepatitis, toxoplasmosis, and abnormal Pap smear.

Treatment:

- Treat <u>asymptomatic</u> patients with CD4 <500, with highly active antiretroviral therapy [HARRT].
- Treat <u>symptomatic</u> patients regardless of CD4 or viral load.
- **Pregnant** patients should be started on HAART despite CD4 count.
- <u>Prophylaxis:</u>
    - CD4 <200 with sulfamethoxazole and trimethoprim (SMP-TMX).
    - CD4 <50 with SMP-TMX and azithromycin (dose once weekly). These medications cover PCP, toxoplasmosis, and *Mycobacterium avium* complex (MAC).

Fun facts:

- Always consider HIV testing for patients with risk factors and non-specific symptoms (diarrhea, rash, or easy bruising).
- Encourage patient to tell sexual partners (in some states, can breach confidentiality to third parties if patient refuses to tell partner/s).
- Human bites more often cause soft tissue infections vs. HIV (saliva does not transmit HIV).
- Do not need to report physicians who have HIV unless conducting activities that could be dangerous to their patients.
- Children with HIV can participate in all sports and attend school with colleagues.
- Do not need to disclose HIV status of child to the school authorities.
- CCR5 mutation is resistant to HIV infection.

- Pregnant women:
    - Should avoid efavirenz in first trimester of pregnancy (can cause neurotube defects).
    - Both mother and baby should receive zidovudine (AZT).
    - Mother should always receive combination HIV therapy.
    - Baby might test false positive shortly after birth, so it is important to test at about 12-18 months to obtain true status. Congenital HIV RNA PCR is the best test.
- HIV medications:
    - AZT can cause thrombocytopenia.
    - Indinavir (inhibits viral protease) can cause crystal-induced nephropathy, which is a well-known side effect. The patient needs to drink lots of water with medication.
    - HAART: goal is to decrease viral load to <50 copies/mL within 6 months.
    - HAART: if develop hyperlipidemia, do not stop medications (if needed); instead, add a statin medication.
    - If patient is not on HAART medications, they should be monitored for CD4 and viral load every 4 months.
    - HIV monotherapy is never used.
    - Needle stick or high-risk exposure from an HIV patient: obtain baseline HIV testing and prophylaxis with lamivudine, AZT, and lopinavir/ritonavir (triple drug therapy) for 4 weeks. Repeat HIV testing in 6 weeks, 12 weeks, and 6 months after exposure. Always wash area with soap, water, and alcohol-based solution.
- Vaccinations in HIV patients:
- IM influenza (annually) and Pneumovax (every 5 years) or if CD4 <200.
- Do not administer live vaccination such as Bacillus Calmette-Guérin. However, it is recommended to administer MMR, which is a live vaccination.

Note: important to remember to monitor viral load and CD4+ count in asymptomatic patients every 4 months (three times a year).

HIV-related infections

Pneumocystis jiroveci pneumonia (PJP)

More commonly seen in patients with AIDs (CD4 <200) and immunodeficient patients. Can present with "bad hypoxia". PJP is an opportunistic infection and not commonly found in healthy individuals.

Hx/PE: Non-productive cough, dyspnea, low-grade fever, and impaired oxygenation.

Diagnosis:

- Best initial test is chest radiography: bilateral interstitial infiltrates with "ground glass" appearance.
- Obtain ABG (very important), sputum culture (very specific especially if CD4 <200), or fiberoptic bronchoscopy with bronchoalveolar lavage (most accurate) with silver stain and immunofluorescence.
- Check viral load (high) and CD4 count (low).

Treatment:

- If PaO2 >70 mmHg, can administer oral SMP-TMX (21 days).
- If PaO2 <70 mmHg, administer high dose IV SMP-TMX and prednisone (taper for moderate to severe hypoxemia).
- Alternative medication is **pentamidine.**
- Discontinue prophylaxis when CD4 >200 for at least 3 months.

Prophylaxis: If CD4 <200 give oral SMP-TMX and folic acid (SMP-TMX can decrease folic acid).

Toxoplasmosis

Toxoplasmosis is a parasitic disease. Usually appears when CD4 <100 and can be contributed to parasites found in raw undercooked meat or cat litter, more common in France. Consult pregnant women on prevention.

Hx/PE: Encephalitis (AIDS patients), altered mental status, seizures, and focal neurologic deficits.

Diagnosis:

- Best initial test is head CT scan (multiple isodense or hypodense "ring-enhancing masses").
- Can detect in blood, amniotic fluid, or cerebrospinal fluid using PCR.
- Repeat head CT scan a few weeks after initiating treatment for resolution.

Note:

- Head MRI findings may appear similar to CNS lymphoma (look for ring-enhancing lesion with mass effect in CNS lymphoma).
- CNS lymphoma needs to be ruled out when standard treatment for toxoplasmosis has failed.
- CNS lymphoma survival rate is determined on degree of immunosuppression.

Treatment:

- High-dose oral pyrimethamine + sulfadiazine with leucovorin for 2 weeks; followed by low doses until clinically resolves or resolves on head CT scan.
- If no improvement after 14 days of treatment, rule out CNS lymphoma, which will require brain biopsy for diagnosis.

Prophylaxis with SMP-TMX (Bactrim DS) if CD4+ <100. Add folic acid with chronic use of SMP-TMX.

Mycobacterium avium complex (MAC)

Causes atypical bacterial infections.

➤ Primary: healthy non-smokers.
➤ Secondary: preexisting pulmonary disease.
➤ Disseminated: common in HIV patients with CD4 <50.

Hx/PE: Weight loss, fatigue, lymphadenopathy, and adrenal insufficiency (if disseminated into adrenals).

Diagnosis:

- CBC (anemia), elevated alkaline phosphatase, and LDH.
- Mycobacterial blood culture, should be performed in individuals with symptoms.

Treatment: At least two agents: clarithromycin and ethambutol plus HAART.

Prophylaxis: start azithromycin if CD4 <50.

Cytomegalovirus (CMV)

A common virus in the same family as herpes virus that can infect both ill and healthy patients. Usually asymptomatic in healthy individuals.

Transmissions: via blood transfusion, sexual contact, breast milk, and respiratory droplets.

Hx/PE: Symptoms will depend on location: for exam, blurry vision (consider CMV retinitis).

- **CMV retinitis**: retinal detachment and hemorrhage.
- **CMV pneumonitis**: common in hematologic malignancies and transplant patients.
- **CMV colitis**: causes urgency, tenesmus, bloody diarrhea, LLQ pain, mucosal ulcers, and hemorrhage.
- **CMV encephalitis**: affects the periventricular region.
- **CMV adrenal insufficiency**: will decrease adrenal-producing hormones.

Diagnosis: PCR (virus isolation, culture, or serum). Negative monospot test.

Treatment:

- Ganciclovir or foscarnet.
- If adrenal insufficiency, will need glucocorticoids and mineralocorticoids.

Progressive multifocal leukoencephalopathy (PML)

Caused by *JC virus* and transmission is unknown. More common in immunosuppressed or HIV patients.

Hx/PE: Gradual symptoms with focal neurological abnormalities such as ataxia, diplopia, and altered mental status.

Diagnosis:

- Best initial test is head CT scan (patchy hypodense lesions in white matter with no edema).
- Head MRI: "non-enhancing" or "no mass effect."
- Obtain viral load and CD4 count.

Treatment: No cure other than HAART.

Note:

- Toxoplasmosis is characterized by "ring enhancing."
- Without HAART treatment, PML patients usually die within 3–6 months.

Tuberculosis (TB)

The main cause of TB is *Myobacterium tuberculosis*. Primary infection is usually asymptomatic and generally affects the lungs, but any organ can potentially be involved, especially in HIV patients.

Risk factors: HIV, alcoholism, immunosuppression, older age, health care work, prison, dorm, and homelessness.

Hx/PE: Non-productive or productive cough, ± hemoptysis, night sweats, chills, and weight loss.

Diagnosis:

- For screening work-up, use PPD skin test.
    - If positive PPD, next step is to confirm with chest radiography.
- Best initial test is chest radiography (this is different from the

screening test, which is PPD).
- Most common finding is upper lobe with cavitation. However, primary infection can be in lower lobe.
- If positive chest radiography, next best step is to obtain a 3:00 am sputum microscopy culture on three separate occasions.
    - Sputum culture with acid-fast test and "red snapper appearance" (gold standard).
    - Three negative sputum cultures are considered non-infectious.
- If sputum cultures are negative and with continued suspicion, perform bronchoscopy with biopsy or bronchoalveolar lavage.
- **Interferon gamma release assay** (IGRA) is more specific than PPD for detecting latent tuberculosis.

Post-exposure: staff in direct contact with patients with tuberculosis (assisted in intubation of a patient) will need PPD testing. If the initial PPD test is negative after exposure, then repeat PPD in 3 months.

Note:
- Patients who have completed appropriate treatment for latent TB do not need a repeat PPD, as this will remain positive long after treatment. Once PPD is positive, the test should never be repeated.
- PPD can be false negative (meaning actually have TB) when CD4 levels <500, which will need to be confirmed with a sputum acid-fast test.
- Rule out HIV in newly diagnosed TB patients (need patients consent).

Positive PPD test:
- >5 mm induration: HIV patients, steroid users, or those in close contact.
- >10 mm induration: indigent people, homeless people, health care workers, residents of a developing nation, and IV drug users.
- >15 mm induration: everyone else.

Note: PPD is read as the greatest area of "induration," not erythema. Erythema often extends beyond the region of induration.

Treatment:
- Active infection: INH, rifampin, pyrazinamide, and ethambutol (2 months), followed by INH and rifampin (4 months). Add vitamin B6 to decrease peripheral neuropathy. Total treatment for 6 months.
- If organism is resistant to INH, can choose a plan with an INH-sparing regimen.
- TB meningitis: INH, rifampin, ethambutol, pyrazinamide, and prednisone (reduce mortality) for 9 months.
- Neonate TB meningitis: treat for about 12 months.
- Latent: example close contact with positive PPD without symptoms or negative chest radiography. Basically, positive PPD with negative chest radiography.
  - Give INH (9 months) plus pyridoxine.
  - If INH resistant then give rifampin for 6 months.
- Pregnant women can be treated with a triple therapy anti-tuberculosis regimen.
  - No streptomycin or pyrazinamide should be administered to pregnant patients.

Note:

✓ If patient wants to leave the hospital without treatment involuntary commitment by court order may be justified.

✓ Health care workers who have been exposed to TB should be tested for baseline PPD at time of exposure and again in 3 months.

✓ Can also restrain with bacterial meningitis secondary to *N. meningococcal*.

Side effects of TB medications:
- Rifampin (revs up P-450, hepatotoxic, and red-orange urine, serum, sweat, tears, and feces).
- Ethambutol (optic neuritis, which presents as painful visual loss and affects red-green discrimination).
- INH (hepatic toxicity and peripheral neuropathy). Can decrease B6 (pyridoxine) and B3 (niacin) levels.

- Pyrazinamide (hyperuricemia, GI intolerance, and *__teratogenic__).
- Streptomycin (nephrotoxicity, ototoxicity, and *__teratogenicity__).

Note: all TB medications can cause liver toxicity (check monthly LFT levels) and should be stopped once transaminases reach approximately 5 times the upper limit of the normal range.

Cryptococcal meningitis

A fungal infection caused primarily from pigeon droppings and can be associated with AIDS (low CD4 cells) and immunosuppressed patients.

Hx/PE: "Absence of meningismus" and presents with mild fever, headaches, and altered mental status.

Diagnosis:

- Lumbar puncture: decreased glucose, increased proteins, increased leukocytosis, and increased pressure.
  - Best initial test: **India ink** (sensitive in approximately 70%).
  - Most accurate test: fungal culture from CSF, serum and urine for **cryptococcal antigen** (95% specific).

Treatment:

- IV amphotericin B <u>plus</u> oral 5-flucytosine for 2 weeks, and then start fluconazole for 2 months.
- Increased intracranial pressure: Patient might need serial lumbar punctures or ventriculoperitoneal (VP) shunts.

Oropharyngeal candidiasis

More commonly seen in patients who are immunosuppressed and/or use antibiotics, corticosteroid inhalers, and dentures.

Hx/PE: Soft white plaques that can be rubbed off easily. Partially raised lesions with a "cottage cheese-like" appearance. Rule out oral hairy leukoplakia (caused by EBV), in which, white plaques cannot be scraped off easily.

Diagnosis:

- Swab back of throat with sterile cotton and examine with KOH slide (budding yeast or pseudohyphae).
- Rule out HIV, unless obvious reason for infection.

Treatment:

- Oral candida: nystatin oral swish (nystatin suspension) or oral fluconazole.
- Candida esophagitis: oral fluconazole.
- Oral hairy leukoplakia: rule out HIV.

Note: remove dentures for 2 weeks. If lesions do not go away, will need biopsy.

Coccidioidomycosis

Also known as, San Joaquin Valley fever, a fungal infection predominant in the "southwest" including California, New Mexico, and Arizona. Infection can involve extrapulmonary sites (most commonly the skin).

Risk factors: immunosuppression, HIV, and pregnancy. Can also happen in non-immunosuppressed patients.

Hx/PE: Mild fever, flu-like symptoms, dry cough, arthralgias, night sweats, erythema multiforme, and erythema nodosum. Basically flu-like symptoms with skin manifestations.

Diagnosis:

- Chest radiography: bilateral infiltrates, bilateral hilar adenopathy, or pleural effusion.
- Sputum culture (dimorphic fungus).
- Bronchoalveolar lavage (if sputum culture not diagnostic).

Treatment:

- Can commonly be self-limiting.
- If patient is pregnant or immunosuppressed, administer treatment.
- Mild: itraconazole or fluconazole (better choice).
- Severe/disseminated/immunosuppressed: IV amphotericin B.

Note: can apply IV amphotericin B followed by a long course of itraconazole.

Blastomycosis

More predominant in the "east coast" and associated with soils and rotten wood. Manifests as a primary lung infection in about 70% of cases and can cause ulcerated skin lesions and lytic bone lesions. The patient does not need to be immunosuppressed.

Hx/PE: flu-like symptoms and lung manifestations along with a rash (papules and pustules that can ulcerate).

Diagnosis:

- Chest radiography: bilateral infiltrates or might resemble tuberculosis findings.
- Sputum culture: KOH (large single "broad budding yeast").
- Most accurate: bronchoalveolar lavage.

Treatment:

- Mild cases: itraconazole.
- Severe cases (severe skin conditions and immunosuppressed patients): amphotericin B.

Note: fluconazole has better CNS penetration than itraconazole.

Histoplasmosis

Fungal infection caused by Histoplasma capsulatum, more common in "Mississippi or Ohio River valley," found in bird and bat droppings.

Hx/PE: Possible fulminant disease, flu-like illness, non-productive cough, fever, weight loss, and lymphadenopathy. Often presents as asymptomatic.

Diagnosis:

- Chest radiography: diffused nodular, cavitary lesions, focal infiltrates, or hilar lymphadenopathy.
- Sputum culture (specific) <u>or</u> culture from the location of the source.

- Bronchoalveolar lavage.
- Urine and serum **polysaccharide antigen test** (sensitive) used for diagnosis and to monitor therapy.

Note: yeast of histoplasmosis can be seen on silver stain.

Treatment:
- Immunocompetent individuals: supportive treatment as often resolves without any treatment.
- Chronic (cavitary lesion): oral itraconazole for ≥1 year.
- Severe or disseminated: amphotericin B.

Aspergillus

Aspergillus is a member of the Ascomycetes fungi that is commonly diagnosed only in immunocompromised patients. **Aspergilloma** (fungus ball) is a growth that develops in an area of past lung disease or lung scarring.

Hx/PE: Progressive asthma-like symptoms: mild fever, cough, hemoptysis, and wheezing.

Diagnosis:
- CBC with differentials: eosinophilia.
- First, obtain chest radiography: cavity lesions and "halo signs" with "air filled levels."
- Sputum culture: accurate test needed for diagnosis.
- Chest CT scan, as cannot diagnose with chest radiological studies alone.

Note: densely consolidated pulmonary infiltrates can grow rapidly with aspergillus infection.

Treatment:
- **Voriconazole** is becoming the drug of choice for invasive aspergillosis.
    - Side effects: voriconazole can cause visual disturbances and hepatotoxicity.
- Fungus balls are not usually treated (with antifungal medicines)

unless there is bleeding into the lung tissue, in such a case, use surgery plus medicines.
- Allergic aspergillosis use oral steroids, not inhaled steroids (which can actually worsen condition).

Note: amphotericin B (inhibits cell membrane permeability of fungal wall) is less favorable because of nephrotoxicity. Can cause renal failure and <u>low</u> serum levels of potassium and magnesium.

Tick bites

Lyme disease

Borrelia burgdorferi, spirochetes, and ixodes genus. More common with people living in or visiting the Northeast part of the United States. Most common complication of tick bites is actually local infection and inflammation. Look for rash and camping/hiking trip in question stem.

Hx/PE: Fever, rash (target like), fatigue, arthralgias, and myalgias.

- <u>Primary disease</u>: **erythema migrans** ("bull's eye" appearance).
- <u>Secondary disease</u>: bell's palsy (CN-7), meningitis, myocarditis, third-degree heart block, or atrioventricular blocks.
- <u>Tertiary disease:</u> arthritis.

Diagnosis:

- Treat if high suspicion without diagnostic confirmation (ELISA and Western blot).
- <u>Primary disease</u>: primarily a clinical diagnosis (primary disease does not usually appear on diagnostic testing).
- <u>Secondary and tertiary disease</u>: ELISA (sensitive) and Western blot (specific). Here, treatment before diagnostic testing.

Treatment:

- Ticks can be removed using tweezers (if tick is full of blood give one dose of doxycycline).
  - Rule out contraindications for doxycycline.
- Start medication first if high suspicion of Lyme disease despite diagnostic studies.

- Early disease in patients >8 years of age: use oral doxycycline.
- Early disease in children (<8 years), pregnant women, or breastfeeding women: use amoxicillin.
- Advanced disease (CNS or cardiac): ceftriaxone or penicillin G.
- Disseminated disease: IV ceftriaxone regardless of age.

Note:
- ✓ Patients with Lyme disease cannot donate blood for 1 year after proper treatment.
- ✓ Lyme disease has a good prognosis after proper antibiotic treatment.

Rocky Mountain spotted fever (*Rickettsia rickettsii*).

Transmitted to humans through a bite of an infected tick, transferred via American dog tick or Rocky Mountain wood tick in the United States. Rickettsii invades endothelial lining of capillaries and invades small vessel vasculitis. Rash moves centrally from wrist and ankles. Severe disease can cause DIC.

Hx/PE: Altered mental status, fever (>102°F), chills, rash, arthralgias, and myalgias.

Diagnosis:
- CBC (low platelets) and LFTs (elevated).
- Rash biopsy or serology (best and most accurate test) with **indirect immunofluorescence antibody**.

Treatment:
- Start treatment before diagnostic work-up.
- Start IV doxycycline before labs (fatal disease).
- Doxycycline is the choice even for children, despite the side effects; can also consider chloramphenicol.

Sexually transmitted diseases
*For more STD information see *Gynecology In Your Pocket*.

Chlamydia

Chlamydia is a gram-negative obligate intracellular microorganism caused by the bacterium *C. trachomatis*. Is the most common bacterial STD (gram-negative, nongonococcal bacteria) and most common cause of blindness in children.

Complications: Reiter's syndrome, Fitz-Hugh-Curtis syndrome (perihepatic infection/fibrosis), PID, ectopic pregnancy, infertility, and lymphogranuloma venereum (painless).

Hx/PE:

- Women: pelvic inflammatory disease (PID), urethritis, cervicitis, vaginitis, and infertility.
- Men: epididymitis (positive Prehn's sign) and penile discharge.

Diagnosis:

- Urine test with PCR (rapid means).
- Pap smear with vaginal culture with PCR (gold standard).
- Gram stain (elevated PMNs but no bacteria).
- Patients diagnosed with an STD, need to be screened for other STDs.

Treatment:

- Oral azithromycin 1 g (single dose) plus treatment for gonorrhea (IM ceftriaxone).
- In **pregnancy**, recommended to use erythromycin and IM ceftriaxone.
- Alternative treatment is doxycycline 100 mg BID for 7 days plus ceftriaxone.
- If PID secondary to chlamydia, use doxycycline (oral, if mild) for 14 days plus ceftriaxone (single dose).
- If **lymphogranuloma venereum**, will need treatment for 21 days with doxycycline plus azithromycin (basically double dosing for chlamydia).

Prevention:

- Always educate patients about safe sex; chalmydia can be prevented with the use of condoms.
- Post-rape prevention antibiotics: ceftriaxone, azithromycin, and metronidazole (covering trichomoniasis).

Gonorrhea

Caused by the bacterium Neisseria gonorrhoeae, which is a sexually transmitted disease. Is a gram-negative intracellular diplococcus that can affect any site in the reproductive tract. A unique characteristic is can cause tenosynovitis.

Hx/PE: Can cause **disseminated gonococcal infection** (monoarticular septic arthritis) and green-yellow urethral purulent discharge.

Diagnosis:

- Pap smear: Gram stain "diplococcal" or can culture using PCR (gold standard).
- Best test for both chlamydia and gonorrhea is the **nucleic acid amplification test** (NAAT).
- Disseminated gonococcal infection: culture joint fluids and mucosal surfaces such as; rectum, urethra, cervix, and oral cavity.

Treatment:

- IM ceftriaxone (single dose) or oral cefepime (single dose) plus always treat presumptive chlamydia with oral azithromycin 1 g (single dose) or oral doxycycline 100 mg BID for 7 days.
- If **pregnant**, use erythromycin in place of azithromycin.

Prevention: always educate patients about safe sex; gonorrhea can be prevented with the use of condoms.

Syphilis (*Treponema pallidum*)

Sexually transmitted disease caused by Treponema pallidum a spirochete that can cause four different stages of the disease. Syphilis can be transmittable to fetus during pregnancy.

Hx/PE:
- Primary syphilis: **chancre** (hard painless ulcers with raised borders), which takes approximately 3 weeks to appear.
- Secondary syphilis: **condylomata lata** (maculopapular rash on soles and palms).
- Latent syphilis with little to no symptoms.
- Tertiary syphilis: **granulomatous gummas**, neurosyphilis, **tabes dorsalis** "high wide slapping gait," **Argyll Robertson** (pupil does not react to light), dilated aortic root, and aortic regurgitation (early diastolic murmur).
- Congenital syphilis: is transmitted during pregnancy or during birth.

Note:

✓ The VDRL test is not specific, as it can be positive for:

    1) viral-mononucleosis/HSV/HIV,

    2) drugs,

    3) rheumatic fever/rheumatoid arthritis (RA), and

    4) SLE/leprosy.

Diagnosis:
- Screening: VDRL (rapid/cheap) but can have false positives. Therefore, confirm with a confirmatory test before treatment.
- Primary syphilis: dark field (spirochetes).
- Secondary syphilis: RPR and FTA-ABS (sensitive and specific).
- Latent stage: serologic evidence of infection without symptoms of disease.
- TPPA: sensitive and specific plus easier to use.

Note: tertiary syphilis will need further work-up with echocardiogram, CSF analysis (lumbar puncture), and ophthalmic exam.

Treatment:
- Uncomplicated primary and secondary syphilis: single dose of IM benzathine penicillin G (2.4 million units).
  - If patient is allergic to penicillin, can use doxycycline for primary and secondary syphilis.

- Latent infection: IM 2.4 million units benzathine penicillin once weekly for 3 weeks.
- Neurosyphilis: also use penicillin IV q4 hours for 14 days; also desensitization, if allergic to penicillin.
- Pregnancy: use penicillin; however, if patient is allergic to penicillin, then penicillin desensitization must be undertaken.

Note:
- ✓ If patient is allergic to penicillin and <u>not</u> pregnant, can use doxycycline or tetracycline for 14 days.
- ✓ Treatment of syphilis can cause **Jarisch-Herxheimer reaction** (flu-like symptoms). If develops, usually self-limiting but can use aspirin.
- ✓ Tertiary syphilis is not infectious.

Haemophilus ducreyi

STD; gram-negative coccobacillus bacteria.

Hx/PE: Irregular deep <u>painful</u> ulceration/s; well-demarcated, necrotic, and inguinal lymphadenopathy.

Diagnosis: First and best test: swab gram stain culture (gram negative, "**school of fish**").

Treatment: IM ceftriaxone, doxycycline, or oral azithromycin.

Human papillomavirus (condylomata acuminate)

Human papillomavirus is the most common viral STD. Subtypes in about 90% of cases that lead to **condylomata acuminate** (benign) are strains 6 and 11. Strains that can lead to squamous cell cancers are 16, 18, and 31. Condylmata acuminate are <u>not</u> contraindications for vaginal delivery.

Hx/PE: "**Cauliflower**" verrucae with skin color appearance on physical exam.

Diagnosis: Clinical diagnosis, acetic acid analysis, or biopsy.

Treatment:

- Cryotherapy, laser removal, podophyllin, imiquimod, or trichloroacetic acid (preferred by many physicians but requires multiple applications).
- Use trichloroacetic acid for **pregnancies**.

Note:

✓ Imiquimod: can also be used for basal cell carcinoma, squamous cell carcinoma, and actinic keratosis.
- This medication is slower acting but does not cause scarring or pain during or after treatment.

✓ Podophyllin: do <u>not</u> use during pregnancy.

Pelvic inflammatory disease (PID)

Polymicrobial infection of the upper genital tract associated with *Neisseria gonorrhea* (1/3 of cases) and chlamydia (1/3 of cases). PID are adhesions (fibrosis) and can cause bowel obstruction secondary to adhesions in chronic cases. Can develop into a tubo-ovarian abscess.

<u>Risk factors</u>: prior STDs, age <35 years, and multiple sexual partners (biggest risk factor).

Hx/PE: Fever, chills, painful intercourse, uterine tenderness, menstrual disturbances, and purulent cervical discharge.

➢ Positive chandelier sign: cervical motion tenderness (most specific finding on physical examination).

Diagnosis:

- Order urine hCG (best initial test), CBC (elevated WBC can tell you the severity), UA, and ultrasound to rule out pregnancy and tubo-ovarian abscess.
- Cervical culture: wet mount and STD panel with NAAT.
- Laparoscopy if standard treatment does not work.
  - It is the most accurate diagnostic tool but rarely needed.

Treatment:

- If high suspicion, start antibiotics prior to lab results.
- Mild to moderate infection: 1 dose IM ceftriaxone, and oral doxycycline for 14 days +/- metronidazole for 14 days. Usually send home after office treatment.
- Severe infection (unstable): requires hospitalization with IV ceftriaxone and IV doxycycline.
- Surgery might be indicated if drainage of tubo-ovarian/pelvic abscess is required, particularly if the mass persists after antibiotic treatment, abscess is >4 cm, or mass is in the cul-de-sac.

Note:

✓ If patient is infertile (tubes are often damaged), most patients will respond to *in vitro* fertilization.

✓ For PID, do not use a single dose of azithromycin (not enough coverage).

Complications: dyspareunia, adhesions, ectopic pregnancy, abscess, infertility, small bowel obstruction, or Fitz-Hugh-Curtis syndrome (pain in RUQ) associated with perihepatitis.

Genitourinary infections

Urinary tract infections (UTIs)

Escherichia coli (gram-negative) is the most common bacteria. More common in women because shorter urethra.

Risk factors: sexual intercourse, hypoestrogenism, catheters, previous UTI, diabetes, pregnancy, antibiotic use, and abnormal anatomy.

Hx/PE: Dysuria, urgency, frequency, "suprapubic pain," hematuria, and foul-smelling urine.

Diagnosis:

- Clinical diagnosis (based on symptoms alone).
- First initial test: urinalysis (increased leukocytes, esterase, and nitrites).

- Small amounts of protein (<150 mg/day) can be normal. If large amounts, work-up with 24-hour urine protein.
- In complicated cases or if treatment has failed order urine culture (most accurate): clean catch and mid-stream are best.
- Microscopic analysis: pyuria, WBC of >5/hpf or 100,000 CFU/mL.

Note: do not need a urine culture before starting treatment, if positive urinalysis with symptoms.

Treatment:

- <u>Asymptomatic patients:</u> require no treatment, unless patient is a child, pregnant, male, or has genitourinary anomalies. Diabetics and elderly patients do not need treatment for asymptomatic UTIs.
- <u>Uncomplicated patients</u> (with symptoms): outpatient oral SMP-TMX for 3 days, fluoroquinolone for 3 days, or nitrofurantoin for 7 days.
- <u>Complicated patients</u>: outpatient oral treatment with same antibiotic but for 7–14 days.
  - Order urine culture.
- **Pregnancy**: nitrofurantoin or cephalosporin plus monthly urine cultures.
  - It is contraindicated to use SMP-TMX in the first trimester of pregnancy (because it decreases folic acid).
  - Nitrofurantoin contraindicated if renal failure, and patient needs to know medication might turn urine brown/red.
- If two UTI infections in 6 month or 3 UTI infections in one year, can give prophylactic antibiotics continuously or solely postcoital.
- Urosepsis: IV antibiotics.
- Do not place catheter, if no obstruction because introduction can cause a secondary infection.

<u>Prophylaxis</u>:

- Usually use low dose SMP-TMX plus folic acid.
  - Be aware that SMP-TMX can cause hyperkalemia especially in patients with renal failure.

- Cranberry juice consumption might be helpful to decrease bacterial adherence to urinary tract.
- In post-menopausal women with recurrent infection, estrogen replacement therapy has been shown to prevent recurrent infections.
- Catheter-associated UTIs: prevent with intermittent catheterization.
    - Do not administer prophylactic antibiotics for long-term catheter placement.

Note: if plan to use SMP-TMX or fluoroquinolones in young fertile females, than obtain an hCG test.

Pyelonephritis

Inflammation of the kidney with similar pathogens as cystitis (*E. coli*). Patients with pyelonephritis are very ill compared to standard UTIs.

Hx/PE: Higher fever, chills, nausea, vomiting, "flank pain," dysuria, polyuria, frothy smelly urine, and urgency.

Diagnosis:
- The work-up is more detailed compared to standard UTIs: CBC (leukocytosis), electrolytes, urinalysis (nitrates [specific], leukocytes [sensitive], esterase, and WBC cast), urine culture, and urine sediment.
- Blood culture: obtain before starting antibiotics to rule out urosepsis.
- Renal CT scan or ultrasound: not generally, necessary but can be used to rule out obstruction (stones), pathology abnormalities, or no responds to therapy after 3–5 days.
- Measure BUN/Cr ratio before CT scan.

Treatment:
- Obtain cultures (blood and urine) before starting antibiotics.
- Mild: outpatient oral fluoroquinolones for 14 days (first line) and increase fluids.
- Severe: IV antibiotics if serious medical complications, vomiting, systemic symptoms, or pregnancy.

- Regimens for hospitalized pyelonephritis: IV ceftriaxone, IV gentamicin, or IV fluoroquinolones.
- Regimen for **pregnant women**: IV ampicillin and gentamycin.
- IV antibiotics should be revised after culture and sensitivity are available and continued until 24-hours after afebrile and can tolerate oral intake. Can discharge patient home and start patient on oral antibiotics for 14 days.

Note: hospitalize if unable to consume oral hydration, take oral medications, decreased patient compliance, high fever, severely ill, or uncertain diagnosis.

Group A hemolytic streptococcus (GAS)

Streptococcus pyogenes is a common cause of pharyngitis, respiratory infection, and soft tissue infection. Can lead to rheumatic fever.

Group B hemolytic streptococcus (GBS)

Streptococcus agalactiae is normal flora in the gut, vagina, and genital tract. Common cause of UTIs in adults and can cause severe disease in neonates.

Nocardia asteroides

An opportunistic infection found mainly in immunocompromised patients. Can cause a respiratory infection (pneumonia).

Hx/PE: Cough, dyspnea, and fever.

Diagnosis:
- Best initial test: chest radiography.
- Sputum culture: Gram stain (Gram positive, aerobic, and partially acid-fast).

Treatment: Oral SMP-TMX is the treatment of choice.

Actinomyces israelii

A facultative anaerobic bacterium. Patient usually with a history of dental trauma or dental procedure, which leads to oral infection or abscess.

Diagnosis: Gram stain (branching), facultative anaerobics, and may form spores.

Treatment: Penicillin for 6-12 days and possible surgery if extensive disease.

Sepsis

Sepsis

A whole-body response to inflammation, usually secondary to an immune response triggered by infection in the blood stream.

Common etiology:
- Gram-positive shock (*Staphylococci*).
- Gram-negative shock (*E. coli*).
- Neonates (GBS).
- Children (*H. influenzae*).
- IV drugs (*S. aureus*).
- Asplenic patients (pneumococcus).

Types:
- **Systemic inflammatory response syndrome (SIRS)**: SIRS is closely related to sepsis, in which patients satisfy criteria for SIRS.
  - **SIRS** = temperature: <36.0°C or >38.0°C; tachypnea: >20 rpm; tachycardia: >90 bpm; and leukocytosis or leukopenia.
- **Severe sepsis**: end-organ dysfunction.
- **Septic shock**: hypotension with organ dysfunction from vasodilation, warm skin, and extremities.

➤ **Cardiogenic shock**: cool skin and extremities.

Hx/PE: Fever, chills, altered mental status, tachycardia, and tachypnea.

Diagnosis: Routine labs: CBC, ESR, CRP, electrolytes, glucose levels, urinalysis, urine culture, blood culture, chest radiography, EKG, sputum culture, and LP (is suspicion).

Treatment: ICU admission, IV fluids (most important step), pressors (if needed), empiric antibiotics, remove catheters and infected lines, and maintain blood pressure to perfuse organs.

Note: most important first step is aggressive fluid resuscitation of at least a CVS of 8–12 mmHg. Add vasopressors if patient is hypotensive or not responding to fluids. Titrated fluids to response of heart rate, blood pressure, and urine output.

Protozoan

Malaria

Disease transmitted by an infected female anopheles mosquito from genus Plasmodium.

Complications: cerebral malaria, severe hemolytic anemia (falciparum), acute tubular necrosis (renal failure) --> "blackwater fever" where hemoglobin are lysed and red blood cells leak into the urine.

Plasmodium types:

    a. Falciparum (has the highest mortality rate, often within 24 hours);
    b. malariae;
    c. vivax, and
    d. ovale.

Hx/PE: Periodic "wax and weaning" symptoms (asymptomatic between attacks), chills, fevers (>41°C), and splenomegaly 4 days after infection.

Diagnosis:

- CBC and MCV might show normochromic-normocytic anemia with elevated reticulocytes.

- Timely diagnosis with **Giemsa stain** or **Wright-stained** thick and thin blood films.
- Determine the strain: PCR (more sensitive study).

Treatment:
- Uncomplicated: orally (treatment depends on strain and if strain resistant to chloroquine).
- *Plasmodium vivax* and *P. ovale*: primaquine is added to chloroquine to eradicate from liver.
- Severe infections: IV quinidine or malarone (a new combination medication).
- Doxycycline is an alternative (100 mg at start of vacation and 4 weeks after departure from malaria area is recommended).

Chemoprophylaxis:
- Mefloquine is recommended in chloroquine-resistant malaria areas such as Africa.
- Chloroquine-sensitive countries are Mexico, Costa Rica, El Salvador, and the Caribbean.
- Atovaquone-proguanil prophylaxis if the patient travels to Brazil.

Animal bites

Rabies

A viral disease that causes inflammation of the brain and caused by mammal bites (most commonly dogs). Rabies is a life-threatening infection and can be fatal once patient is symptomatic. Latency can be weeks to years before onset of symptoms.

Hx/PE: Fever, AMS, violent movements, and uncontrolled excitement.

Diagnosis:
- Fluorescent antibody test or PCR.
- Cerebral inclusion bodies called **Negri bodies** are 100% diagnostic.

Treatment:
- <u>Wild animal</u>:
  - If <u>not</u> previously vaccinated: then give 4 doses of vaccine plus 1 dose of immunoglobulin.
  - If previously vaccinated: then give 2 doses of rabies vaccination.
- <u>Domestic animal</u>: observation of animal for 10 days. No treatment if normal behavior in animal.
- <u>Sick animal</u>: biopsy brain of animal.
  - <u>If negative</u>: no treatment.
  - <u>If positive</u>: if not previously vaccinated then 4 doses of vaccination (day 0, 3, 7, and 14) plus 1 dose of immunoglobulin. If previously vaccinated then give 2 doses of rabies vaccination (day 0 and 3).

Note:
- ✓ As a rule of thumb, if history of recent vaccination, patient will need a booster vaccination <u>only</u>.
- ✓ If <u>no</u> history of vaccination, will need both immunoglobulin and vaccinations.

Ocular infections

*Inflammation of conjunctiva secondary to viral, bacterial, fungal, or parasitic infections.

Bacterial conjunctivitis

Hx/PE: Unilateral, thick purulent discharge, normal vision, no itchiness, and with a foreign body sensation.

Diagnosis: Clinical diagnosis or Gram stain culture, if not treated by standard treatment.

Treatment:
- Is usually self-limiting (1-2 weeks).
- Topical antibiotic drops: erythromycin or sulfa drops.

- Fluoroquinolones (ciprofloxacin) should be used in contact wearers (*Pseudomonas*). Also important to tell patient to stop wearing contact lens.
- Can return to school or work 24 hours after starting treatment.

Note: topical steroids are <u>not</u> used in bacterial corneal ulceration because of possible spread and worsening of the condition.

Viral conjunctivitis

Adenovirus most common. If secondary to herpes virus, look for "dendritic ulcers."

Hx/PE: Bilateral watery discharge, itchy, and severe ocular irritation.

Diagnosis: Clinical diagnosis. If foreign body sensation, rule out corneal abrasive damage with fluorescein slit-lamp.

Treatment:

- Contagious but self-limiting; wash hands frequently and good hygiene.
- Antihistamine, cold compresses, and lubricants may be used to help with the symptoms.
- If secondary to herpes virus, can use oral acyclovir (optic 3% acyclovir gel not as useful).
- Severe (topical corticosteroids): supervision by ophthalmologist.

Prevention: avoid sharing towels, linens, and cosmetics.

Neisseria gonorrhoeae conjunctivitis

Medical emergency that can lead to blindness. Usually presents around day 3 post-partum.

Diagnosis: Gram stain (diplococcal) or PCR.

Treatment:

- IM ceftriaxone or oral ciprofloxacin. Use both oral and topical antibiotics.
- Topical medications are used for prophylaxis at birth.

Chlamydia trachomatis conjunctivitis

Leading cause of blindness, corneal scarring, and "neovascularization." Usually presents around day 7 post-partum.

Diagnosis: Cannot see chlamydia on Gram stain; use Giemsa stain or PCR. Need to rule out chlamydia trachomatis pneumonia.

Treatment: Oral erythromycin (treatment of choice), oral tetracycline, or oral doxycycline. Use both oral and topical antibiotics.

Prevention: topical silver nitrate (1% solution) or erythromycin drops are used as a prophylaxis for ocular chlamydia in newborn infants but not for treatment.

Orbital cellulitis

Medical emergency

Can lead to blindness, common after sinus infection by direct spread via the ethmoid sinus through the lamina. Common bacteria: Streptococci, staphylococci, and *H. influenzae*. If diabetic, consider mucormycosis and rhizopus.

Risk of developing CST.

Hx/PE: Proptosis, ocular pain, decreased extraocular movements, and decreased visual acuity.

Diagnosis: Mostly clinical. Head MRI used to rule out ocular abscess or intracranial involvement.

Treatment:
- Immediate IV antibiotics (emergency, consider treatment before studies) with both penicillins and cephalosporins. Consider other antibiotics to prevent resistant.
- Diabetics with rhizopus (IV amphotericin B).
- Ophthalmological consult.

Corneal abrasion

Damage of the epithelial layer of the cornea, most commonly caused by trauma.

Hx/PE: Painful, photophobia, and "foreign body sensation."

Diagnosis: **Fluorescein slit-lamp** (use topical tetracaine before examination).

Note: herpes ocular infection can mimic corneal abrasion and can be seen on slit-lamp.

Treatment:

- No specific therapy (patching the eye has no clear benefit).
- Can administer empiric broad-spectrum antibiotics eye drops or ointment because of increased risk of staphylococcus infections.

Chalazion

A cyst in the eyelid caused by inflammation.

Hx/PE: Usually painless "rubbery nodule" on eyelid.

Diagnosis: Consider biopsy to rule out cancer (more commonly basal cell carcinoma).

Treatment: Self-limiting (usually within a few months), can apply warm compresses, topical antibiotic eye drops, local steroid injections or surgical removal.

Hordeolum (stye)

Commonly caused by staphylococcus aureus bacterium, which causes an inflammation of the internal or external glands of the eyelid. Most frequent complication of a stye is development into a chalazion.

Risk factors: poor hygiene, dehydration, decreased sleep, and rubbing of eyes.

Hx/PE: Painful or non-painful erythema papule on upper or lower eyelid.

Diagnosis: Clinical diagnosis.

Treatment: Antibiotics (erythromycin ophthalmic ointment) and hot compresses. Surgical drainage on rare occasions.

Endocarditis

Infective endocarditis (IE)

An inflammation of the endocardium, which can involve damage of heart valves. The inflammation causes a lack of blood supply to the valves, leaving them susceptible to infections and low circulation of antibiotics to the area.

Etiology:

- *S. aureus* → IV drugs.
- *S. epidermidis* → prosthetic valve.
- Candida → indwelling catheters.
- Viridans → dental procedure.
- *S. bovis* → GI malignancy.
- SLE → Libman-Sacks endocarditis.

Types:

➢ **Acute endocarditis**: commonly caused by *S. aureus*, faster onset, about 30–40% of cases, and causes right side heart pathology.

➢ **Subacute endocarditis**: commonly caused by viridans, slower onset, about 40–60% of cases, causes left side heart pathology.

Hx/PE: "FROM JANE" <u>f</u>ever, **R**oth spots (retinal hemorrhages), **O**sler's nodes (nodules on finger and toes), <u>m</u>urmurs, **J**aneway lesions (nontender maculae on the palms and soles), <u>a</u>nemia, <u>n</u>ail bed hemorrhages, and <u>e</u>mboli. Can have glomerulonephritis.

Diagnosis:

- CBC: leukocytosis with left shift and increased ESR and CRP.
- Blood culture (rule out sepsis) --> obtain before starting antibiotics.
- Echocardiogram (new murmurs):
    - Transesophageal echocardiogram (TEE) is more specific than transthoracic echocardiogram (TTE) for evaluating the degree of damage or destruction of valves.
    - If valvular damage, will need a cardiac surgery consult.
- Diagnosis based on **Duke's criteria** (1 major and 2 minor <u>or</u> 2 major and 1 minor).

- Major criteria include positive blood culture and positive endocardiogram.

Treatment:
- Start antibiotics immediately if highly suspected.
- Standard treatment is vancomycin (4–6 weeks) and gentamicin (2 weeks).
- IV antibiotics: vancomycin <u>or</u> nafcillin + gentamicin <u>or</u> ceftriaxone + ampicillin/sulbactam.
- Surgical valve replacement has a low threshold with ejection fraction <60% including symptoms of orthopnea or dyspnea.
- Will need eye exam and echocardiogram monitoring.

<u>Prophylactic antibiotics:</u> oral amoxicillin (use macrolides if allergic) 1 hour before dental procedures with previous endocarditis, prosthetic valves, or unrepaired congenital heart disease (cyanotic type); exceptions are ASD and VSD, which do <u>not</u> need prophylaxis.

Fun facts:
- ✓ Corticosteroids can be potentially fatal (NEVER use here).
- ✓ If infusion of vancomycin and presents with **red man syndrome** (release of histamine), slow the infusion of vancomycin.
- ✓ If <u>rash</u> allergy with use of penicillin, can use cephalexin.
- ✓ If <u>anaphylaxis</u> allergy with use of penicillin, can use azithromycin.

Osteomyelitis

Osteomyelitis

Bone infection and inflammation more commonly seen in trauma, peripheral artery disease, and diabetic patients.

<u>Common pathogens:</u>
- ➢ *S. aureus* (most common overall).
- ➢ IV drug user → *S. aureus*.
- ➢ Sickle cell disease → salmonella.
- ➢ Surgery → *S. epidermidis*.

- Foot puncture → *pseudomonas*.
- Diabetic → polymicrobial and *pseudomonas*.
- Sexually active with unprotected sex → gonococcus (history of urethra discharge).

Note: pathology of patient can increase risk of certain infections, but *S. aureus* is the most common despite pathology.

Complications:

- Sepsis, septic arthritis, **marjolin's ulcer** (can lead to squamous cell cancer), osteoarthritis, and infections.
- Nongonococcal (elderly) or gonococcal (usually younger patients).

Hx/PE: Fever, chills, localized bone pain, warmth, swelling, erythema, and limited motion.

- Direct spread: about 80% of the time, more common in adults from soft tissue inflammation and infection, like cellulitis or trauma.
- Hematogenous seeding (blood): about 20% of the time, more common in children. More commonly caused by *S. aureus*.

Diagnosis:

- Best initial test is obtaining a radiograph (often negative or can show periosteal elevation).
- Second test: MRI (specific) is first line for confirmation.
  - However, contraindicated if patient has hardware.
- Most accurate test: bone biopsy and culture.
- CBC: leukocytosis (>50,000/mm³ WBC), elevated ESR (also used to monitor response to treatment), and elevated CRP.
- Blood culture: helpful to rule out sepsis and to identify organism.

Note:

✓ If clinical suspicion of **septic arthritis**, the next best step is arthrocentesis.

✓ Bone scan and MRI have the same sensitivity. However, MRI has a much higher specificity.

Treatment:

- IV antibiotics: most commonly vancomycin and ceftriaxone

for 4–6 weeks. Adjust according to blood cultures and bone biopsy culture.
- Surgical debridement if necrotic <u>or</u> not treated after standard treatment of antibiotics.
- If severe gangrene or sepsis, patient might require amputation.

Note:
✓ Antibiotics alone are often sufficient for children.
✓ In adults, usually need antibiotics <u>plus</u> surgical debridement.

Antibiotic choices:
- **MSSA**: oxacillin/nafcillin <u>or</u> clindamycin + ciprofloxacin + ampicillin/sulbactam.
- **MRSA**: vancomycin and ceftriaxone (gram-negative bacteria). Vancomycin only covers gram-positive bacteria.

Note:
✓ Linezolid, quinupristin, and dalfopristin: anti-staphylococcal agents that are reserved for vancomycin-resistant *S. aureus*.
✓ Renally dose vancomycin and levofloxacin.

Anthrax

Caused by *Bacillus anthracis*, which is a Gram-positive spore forming bacterium. More commonly affects farmers and veterinarians. Also used as a biological weapon

➤ Cutaneous anthrax (most common): pruritic papules with edematous halo around the edges, which become "black eschars," and regional lymphadenopathy.

➤ Inhalation anthrax (most deadly): fever, hypoxia, and pneumonia symptoms with hemorrhagic mediastinitis.

➤ Gastrointestinal anthrax: from uncooked meat; presents with abdominal pain, nausea, vomiting, and bloody stools (necrosis).

Diagnosis:
- Inhalation anthrax: chest radiography, widened mediastinum, and sputum culture with Gram stain.
- Cutaneous or GI anthrax: culture with Gram stain.

- PCR is also helpful in diagnosis.

Treatment: Inhalation or cutaneous: ciprofloxacin or doxycycline, plus add one or two other antibiotics.

Botulinum toxin

Clostridium botulinum is a neurotoxic protein. Also known as its commercial brand name **Botox**. Most commonly caused by ingestion of environmental dust or honey. Patients usually have a complete recovery.

Hx/PE: Constipation and lethargy are usually the first manifestations.

Diagnosis: *C. botulinum* spores or toxins in stool.

Treatment: Give **botulinum antitoxin**, not antibiotics, which will actually increase release of toxins (human-derived botulism immunoglobulin).

Note: infant botulism can inhibit gag reflex, which can cause aspiration.

Index

A

actinomyces israelii 45
acute otitis media 7
acute pharyngitis 9
acute sinusitis 6
anthrax 55
Argyll Robertson 38
aspergillus 33
aspiration pneumonia 4
aspiration pneumonitis 6
atypical bacteria 4
atypical pneumonia 3, 5

B

bacterial conjunctivitis 48
bacterial meningitis 15
bacterial pharyngitis 9
blastomycosis 32
botulinum toxin 56
brain abscess 19
brain herniation 20

C

cavernous sinus thrombosis 20
chalazion 51
chancre 38
chlamydia 36
chlamydia trachomatis conjunctivitis 50
chronic sinusitis 6
citrobacter koseri 17
clindamycin 20
coccidioidomycosis 31
community-acquired pneaumonia 5
community-acquired pneumonia 4
condylomata acuminate 39
condylomata lata 38
corneal abrasion 50
cropharyngeal candidiasis 30
cryptococcal antigen 30
cryptococcal meningitis 30
cystic fibrosis 5
cytomegalovirus 26

D

disseminated gonococcal infection 37
Duke's criteria 52

E

ELISA test 21
encephalitis 18
endocarditis 52
erythema migrans 34

F

fever of unknown origin 15
Fluorescein slit-lamp 51

G

Giemsa stain 47
gonorrhea 37
granulomatous gummas 38
group A hemolytic streptococcus 44
group B hemolytic streptococcus 44

H

haemophilus ducreyi 39
heterophile antibody 13
histoplasmosis 32
HIV 21
HIV-related infections 24
hordeolum 51
hospital-acquired pneumonia 5
human immunodeficiency virus 21
human papillomavirus 39

I

indirect immunofluorescence antibody 35

Index, cont'd.

IgM EBV antibody to viral capsid antigen 13
infectious mononucleosis 12
infective endocarditis 52
influenza 11
interferon gamma release assay 28
intranasal influenza vaccination 12

K

kissing disease 12

L

legionellosis 5
Lyme disease 34
lymphogranuloma venereum 36

M

malaria 46
malignant otitis externa 9
marjolin's ulcer 54
meningitis 14
mononucleosis 12
monospot test 13
MRSA 55
MSSA 55
mycobacterium avium complex 25
myringotomy 8

N

Negri bodies 47
neisseria gonorrhoeae conjunctivitis 49
neonate PNA 5
nocardia asteroides 44

O

orbital cellulitis 50
osteomyelitis 53
otitis externa 8

P

pelvic inflammatory disease 40
peritonsillar abscess 10
pharyngitis 9
pneumocystis jiroveci pneumonia 24
pneumonia 3
polysaccharide antigen test 33
post-viral 5
progressive multifocal leukoencephalopathy 27
protozoan 46
pyelonephritis 43

R

rabies 47
rapid influenza diagnostic test 11
retropharyngeal abscess 11
rickettsia rickettsii 35
Rocky Mountain spotted fever 35

S

San Joaquin Valley fever 31
scarlet fever 14
sepsis 45
septic arthritis, 54
septic shock 45
sinusitis 6
speech and swallow study 6
strawberry tongue 14
stye 51
swimmer's ear 8
syphilis 37
systemic inflammatory response syndrome 45

T

tabes dorsalis 38
TB meningitis 29

Index, cont'd.

tonsillectomy 10
toxoplasmosis 24
Treponema pallidum 37
tuberculosis 27
typical bacteria 4
typical pneumonia 3

U

urinary tract infections 41

V

viral conjunctivitis 49
viral meningitis 15
viral pharyngitis 9
voriconazole 33

W

Western blot 21
Wright-stained 47

www.ingramcontent.com/pod-product-compliance
Lightning Source LLC
Chambersburg PA
CBHW040846180526
45159CB00001B/331